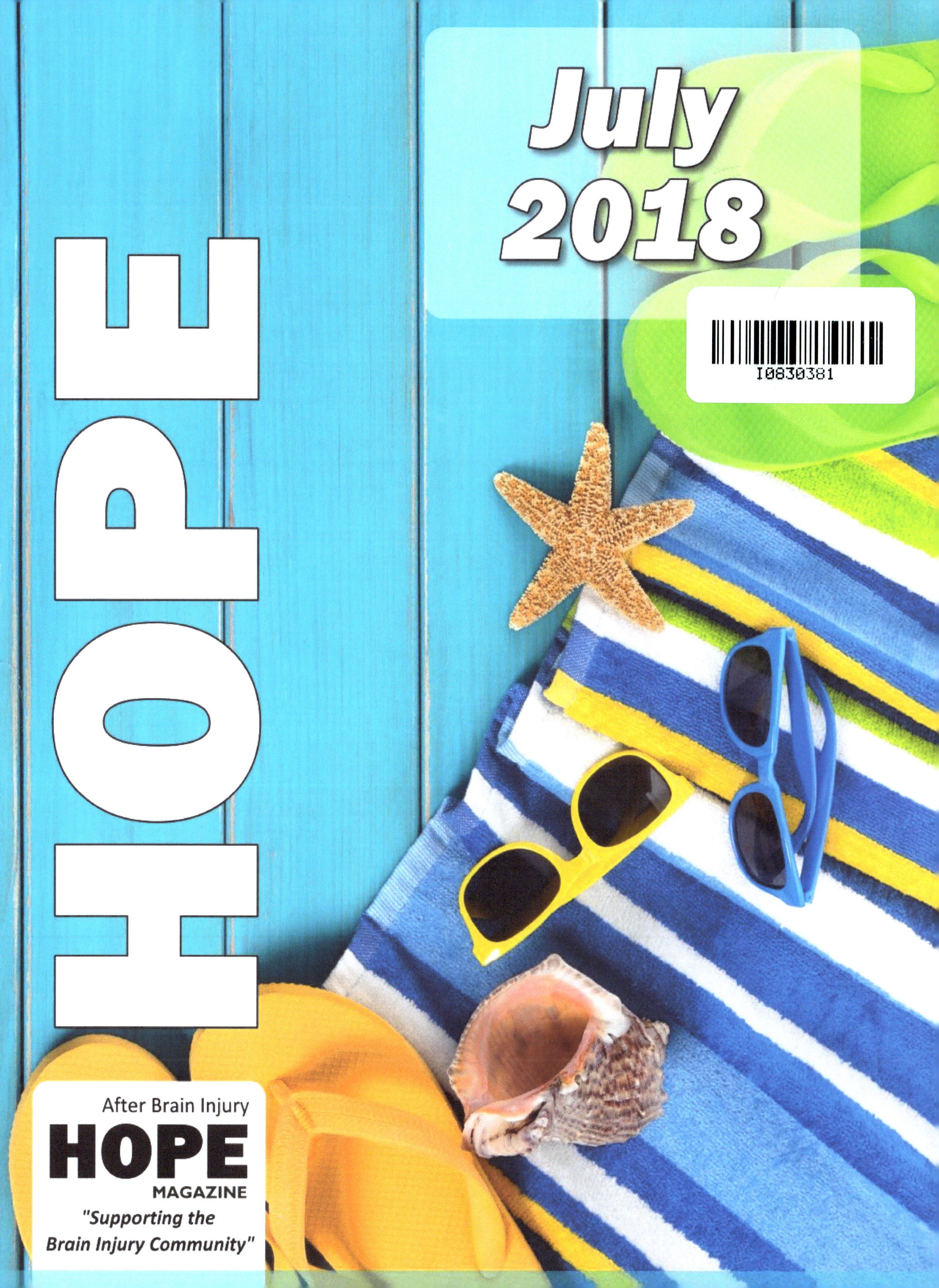

July
2018
I0830381
HOPE
After Brain Injury
HOPE
MAGAZINE
"Supporting the
Brain Injury Community"

Welcome

HOPE MAGAZINE

Serving the Brain Injury Community

July 2018

Publisher
David A. Grant

Editor
Sarah Grant

Contributing Writers

Katy Austin
Ted Baxter
David A. Grant
Tiffany Gross
Christina Riley
Jeff Sebell
Mary Underwood
Lisa Yee

FREE subscriptions at
www.HopeAfterBrainInjury.com

Welcome to the July 2018 issue of HOPE Magazine!

As we move through our fifth year of publication, I continue to be amazed and inspired by the stories shared by our contributors.

Back in 2012, when I sustained my own brain injury, I thought that my life was over. Suffice to say, I was quite wrong.

It seems that I'm not the only one who was wrong. In this month's issue, you will read story after story about survivors who have fought back, steadfastly saying, "This is not how my story is going to end!"

We are also pleased to feature stories from a caregiver's perspective. As those of us within the brain injury community already know, brain injury affects everyone.

Interested in sharing your story? We are always looking for new contributors. You don't need to be a professional writer. In fact, we prefer that you are not.

You can reach out to me personally at david@tbihopeandinspiration.com for more information.

Peace,

David A. Grant
Publisher

Contents

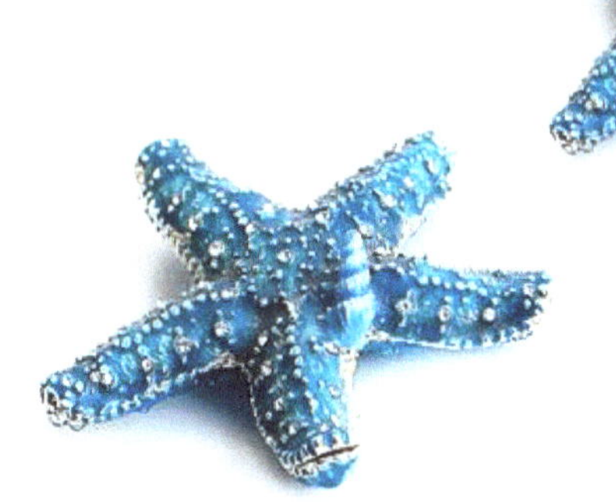

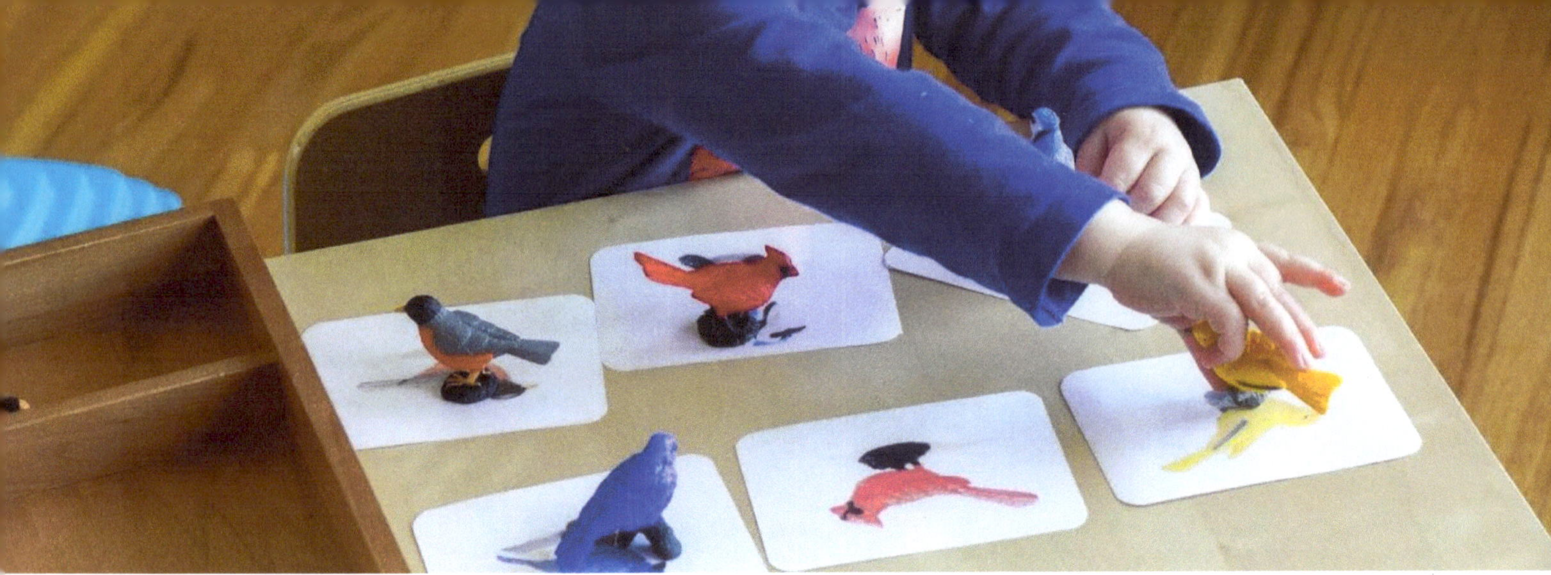

Coming Back From Beyond

By Ted Baxter

Having held the position of global financial executive for a prestigious global investment hedge fund, flying was not a new experience for me. On top of that, there were the exotic vacations I took with my former wife, Kelly. When I wasn't flying for work, I was flying for pleasure. So, perhaps I should have realized right away that the pain in my leg wasn't a result of exhaustion and too much sitting on a plane. It was when Kelly asked me a question and I didn't respond that she realized something was seriously wrong.

I heard her questions and sounds from the paramedics and doctors, but I couldn't comprehend what they were saying. It was almost like having quick flashes of information in my eye, gradual shading of comprehension from one side like a curtain being drawn. I couldn't respond, I couldn't talk, I had a huge headache, and my body was starting to shut down. That sense of clarity abandoned me by the time we arrived at the hospital.

> "I heard her questions and sounds from the paramedics and doctors, but I couldn't comprehend what they were saying."

My blood pressure plummeted well below what was deemed 'low blood pressure' and at one point, fell to 32. I did become lucid again, because I remember choking on a chewable aspirin and being disturbed by the lack of sensation in my arm.

My stroke was caused by a blood clot, a deep vein thrombosis (DVT), in my right shin which travelled to my heart and eventually landed in my brain.

Motivation and Determination

I was transferred from the hospital in Evanston, IL to Rehabilitation Institute of Chicago (RIC) and began working with highly trained physical, speech, and occupational therapists. At the beginning of my stay in RIC, the weekends were quiet with nobody around except the nurses and Kelly. I knew that time is the essence of recovery. Saturdays and Sundays became days when I went to the exercise room down the hall to attempt sit-ups and stretches. Kelly put me in a wheelchair with the aid of the nurses and rolled me into the exercise room.

I continued to struggle to form intelligible words. I couldn't read or write. It took three or four months for me to remember Kelly's name. It was while I was at RIC that I was first introduced to the term "aphasia." I had lost a great deal as a result of the stroke, including my abilities to walk and talk, but I had not lost my will and determination.

By the time I was released from RIC, about two months after having the stroke, I was walking, albeit with a limp, something that most never thought I would do again. As good as that felt, I left the facility aggravated by my aphasia and determined to find a solution. I managed to communicate to Kelly that I wanted her to purchase for me flash cards meant for toddlers. I needed to retrain my brain, and that meant starting at the beginning.

She would hold up pictures of everyday objects and I would fight my way through the words, often attempting numerous times before I could mimic the way Kelly would say them.

A few minutes later, when shown the exact same picture, I would have completely forgotten the associated word. Short-term memory became my biggest foe. But I was determined and I continued my own methods of recovery between sessions with speech therapists at the RIC Outpatient Program.

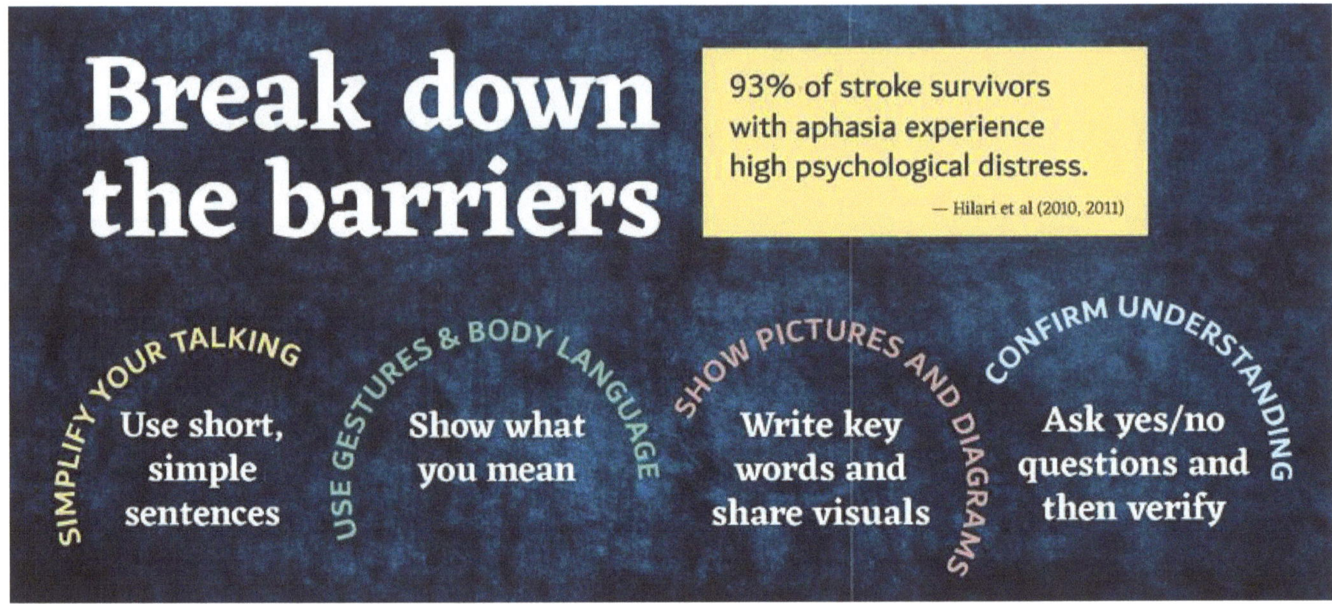

Graphic Source: National Aphasia Association

I found a computer application that featured a woman carefully forming words and I would mimic her sounds and how her mouth moved when the right pronunciation was used. I was given crossword puzzles, which I would do on my lunch break. In my mind, I didn't have time to waste. It might be because of my haste that I found the group therapy sessions so torturous, but I also hated being unable to answer the questions asked. I like to be the best in everything and aphasia was robbing me of that ability. I didn't have the words yet, but I had my memories and I knew that I had given speeches at important international conferences, did impromptu pep-talk speeches to my employees, and interacted with businessmen from all over the world.

Aphasia Training in Ann Arbor

Kelly was always trying to learn more. She did research into other programs in the country and discovered the University of Michigan Aphasia Program (UMAP). I willingly made the trek from Chicago to Ann Arbor to enroll in UMAP. During my first conversation with the speech therapist, she told me that it was very clear that I wasn't always comprehending what others were saying to me. That was an eye-opening moment for me. I knew that I had trouble speaking sensibly, but I hadn't realized that I was confusing what others were trying to communicate to me.

The therapists at UMAP really tried to cater to my specific needs. In one session, the primary speech therapist pulled out the financial page of the *Wall Street Journal* and proceeded to ask me questions related to the financial world that I had once lived in. This jogged my memory to know terms I had used frequently before my stroke. This became a regular part of the therapy routine, with her challenging me to relearn the familiar terms.

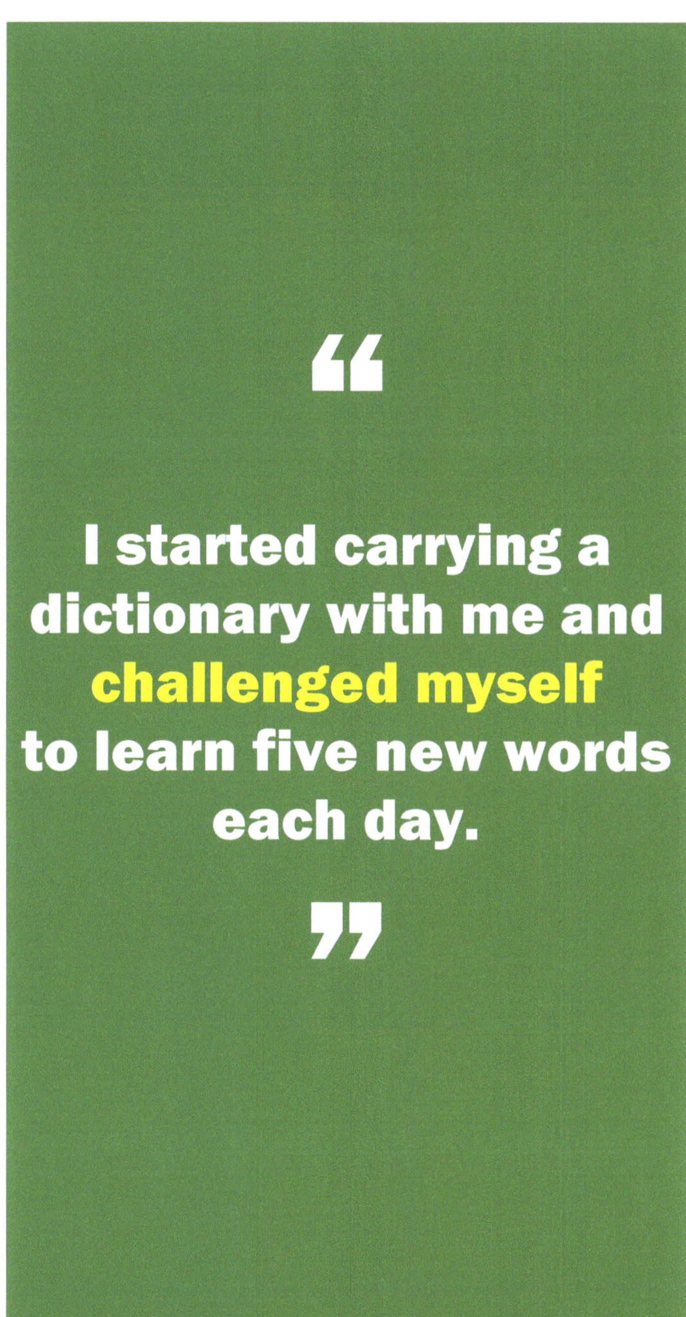

Variety of Activities to Avoid Boredom

Frustrated but determined, I did simple things like practicing writing my name twenty times every day and trying to speak clearly and fluently using a tape recorder of my voice. I then went back to a deck of flashcards and started practicing using a different form. I read the question on one side and then flipped it over and read the answer on the other. My goal was to recall what I had read. *Practice, practice, practice!!!*

I participated in a speech program at Northwestern University in Evanston, IL. While I was there, I was encouraged to consider participating in a book club, which I agreed to try. Each week, we were assigned a few pages of the designated book to read, and clinicians would ask us follow up questions. I changed the rules for myself, though, and made it a goal to ask at least two comprehension-based queries every week. If I could do that, it meant that I was really understanding what I was reading. Around this time, I started carrying a dictionary with me and challenged myself to learn five new words each day. That meant not only reading and understanding them, but also using them in sentences throughout the day and writing them out on flashcards.

This provided me an atmosphere where part of the speech program involved working with doctoral students, completing a variety of different tasks. They would show me pictures of people doing activities, speak the corresponding verb, and then ask me to use the word in a sentence. I really enjoyed this, and it was very beneficial to my recovery. The accomplishments were great self-esteem boosters.

Recovery Moved to A Change in Perspective

After I had spoken to a variety of people, some friends and some strangers, I decided that I needed a change.

In 2010, I moved to Southern California, even though I knew no one there. All of my life, I had been a risk-taker, so I took a chance. I was scared, but I had never let fear stop me before. Slowly but surely, I volunteered myself to the hospitals near where I lived. I was introduced to several medical doctors at the University of California – Irvine, and I attended a speech program at San Diego State University. I took it upon myself to make connections going forward.

Today, I am involved in a volunteer communication recovery group at St. Jude's Hospital, where I provide therapy to stroke survivors and train students to be better clinicians. I'm involved in philanthropic matters of UC Irvine - Health, and I'm a member of the Board of Directors of the American Heart and Stroke Association in Orange County.

I wrote my memoir, *Relentless: How a Massive Stroke Changed My Life For The Better,* which will be published in July of 2018.

It would have been much easier to have given in to the effects of the stroke and to admit defeat to aphasia, but it is so much more rewarding to know that I did what so many believed I wouldn't be able to do.

Meet Ted Baxter

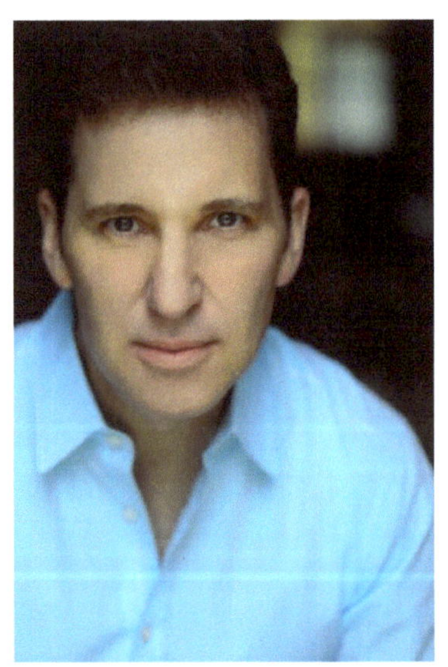

After spending 22 years in the financial industry, Ted W. Baxter retired as a global finance executive with a large hedge investment firm based in Chicago. Ted now resides in Newport Beach, CA where he volunteers at several health-related institutions and hospitals in Orange County, leading groups in a stroke-related communication recovery program and is a member of the Board of Directors at the American Heart and Stroke Association. He is the author of "Relentless: How A Massive Stroke Changed My Life for the Better." For additional information about Ted, please visit www.tedwbaxter.com.

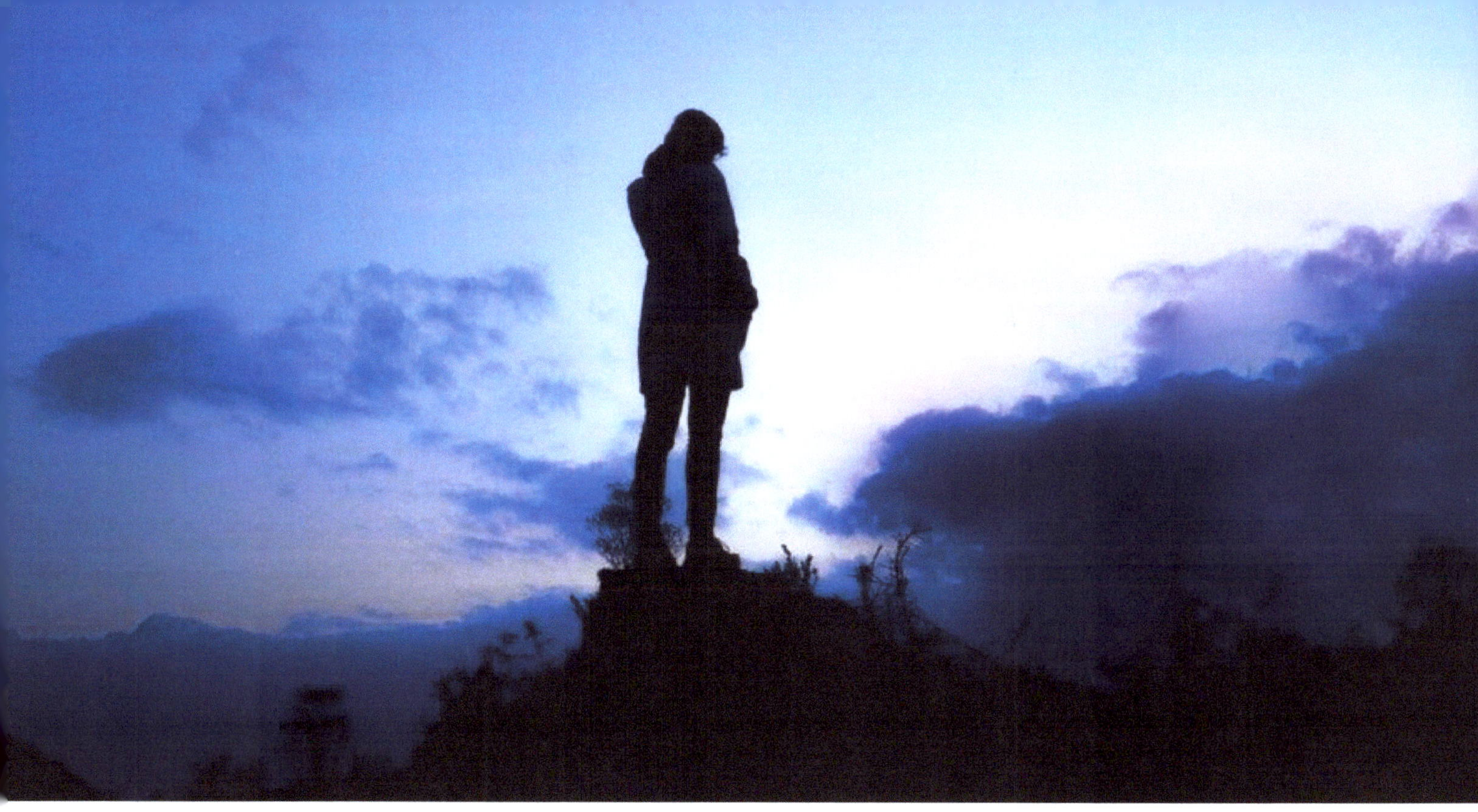

Rocky

By Lisa Yee

Just over a mile from our house stands an improbably high hill topped by a graffiti-covered boulder in the shade of an oak tree. Back in my pre-brain injury days a decade ago, I'd get up early and go for a run before work, ending it with the zigzagging uphill terrain of what I called the Mountain.

I also had a name for the boulder: Rocky, which I'd then sit on to catch my breath and take in the glorious view. There was a pristine lake surrounded by a walking/cycling path that was in turn surrounded by Forest Preserve woodlands and trails. And at that hour, there were no people.

After a while, I'd walk downhill and back home to start my day. At the time, I was a regional editor at a suburban Chicago newspaper, so my job involved a lot of sitting in my office, typing and fretting—pretty much like any occupation, now that I think about it.

Those early morning runs energized me for more than work. There was also the usual stuff of life— housework, grocery shopping, cooking (mostly prep work for my husband, the real cook), and shuttling our daughter between school and gymnastics.

It was on one of those nights after gymnastics practice that The Accident changed our lives. I drove to the gym and let our daughter, who was then fifteen and had her learner's permit, drive us home. At a four-way stop three blocks from our house, there was a crash. I have no memory of any of this, of course.

Thank God, I was the only one injured.

I was airlifted to a Trauma 1 hospital in Chicago. Besides moderate traumatic brain injury and acquired epilepsy, I'd suffered a fractured pelvis and five other broken bones, a lacerated liver, a bruised lung and two cracked teeth. I didn't regain consciousness for a week.

I awoke remembering my daughter as the skinny middle school girl with braces she once was. Now, it was jolting to see the high school beauty she'd become.

During the time I was in a coma, my husband had plastered my hospital room walls with photos and mementos from different periods in our lives, in the hope that they would help me recover memories. He'd printed out a saying from Mali that was told to him by my sister, who had served there in the Peace Corps: "*Dooni dooni kononi be nyaga da*," which translates to "Little by little, the bird builds its nest." In other words, we may not see progress all at once, but with persistence and patience, we'll get there.

I still have that sign.

He had also gone to my favorite running destination, Rocky, and taken a photo for my wall. For him, Rocky had come to symbolize my uphill climb to come back, to remember, to recover.

After my release from the hospital and long physical recovery at the rehab center and at home, my husband and I walked together up the Mountain. I climbed the

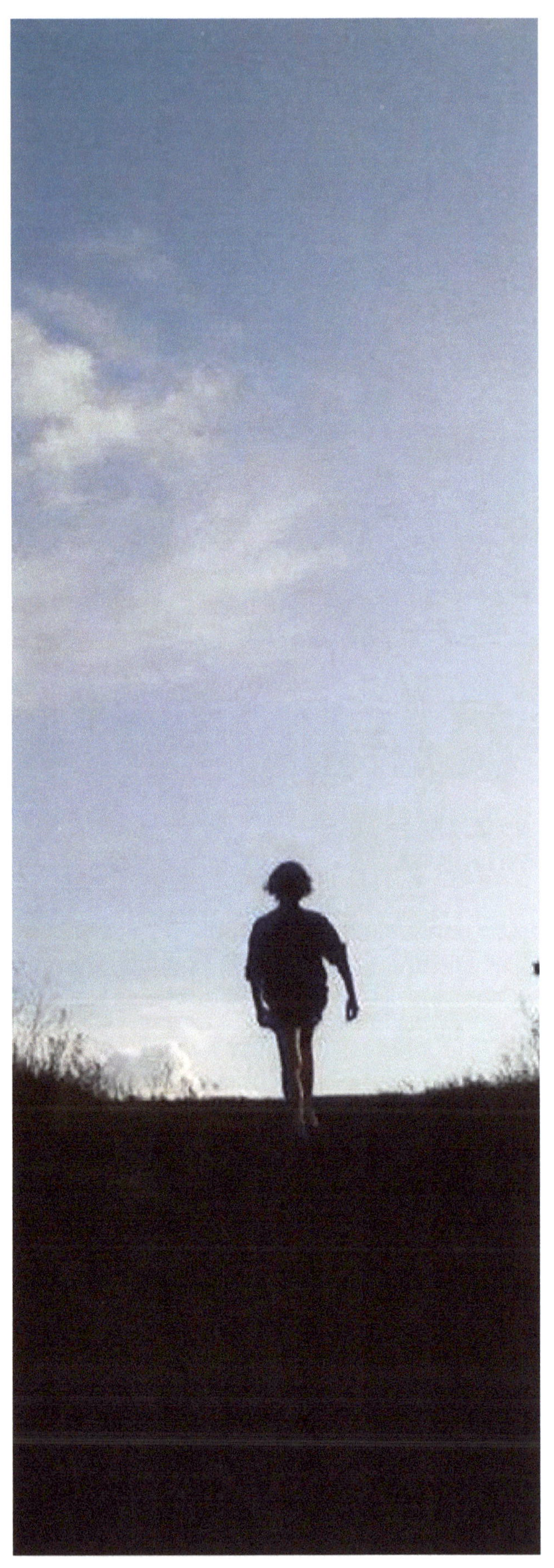

topmost section myself while he photographed me from behind as I reached the summit. The photo shoot continued as I turned and raised my arms in triumph.

Eventually I returned to running, although the Rocky area was off limits unless someone came with me, because of its remoteness. I soon was running 5K races again and even did a 10K.

Those were good years. But now it seems my brain won't let me do what I love. During several runs and races I started having seizures, and sometimes ambulances hauled me off to the hospital.

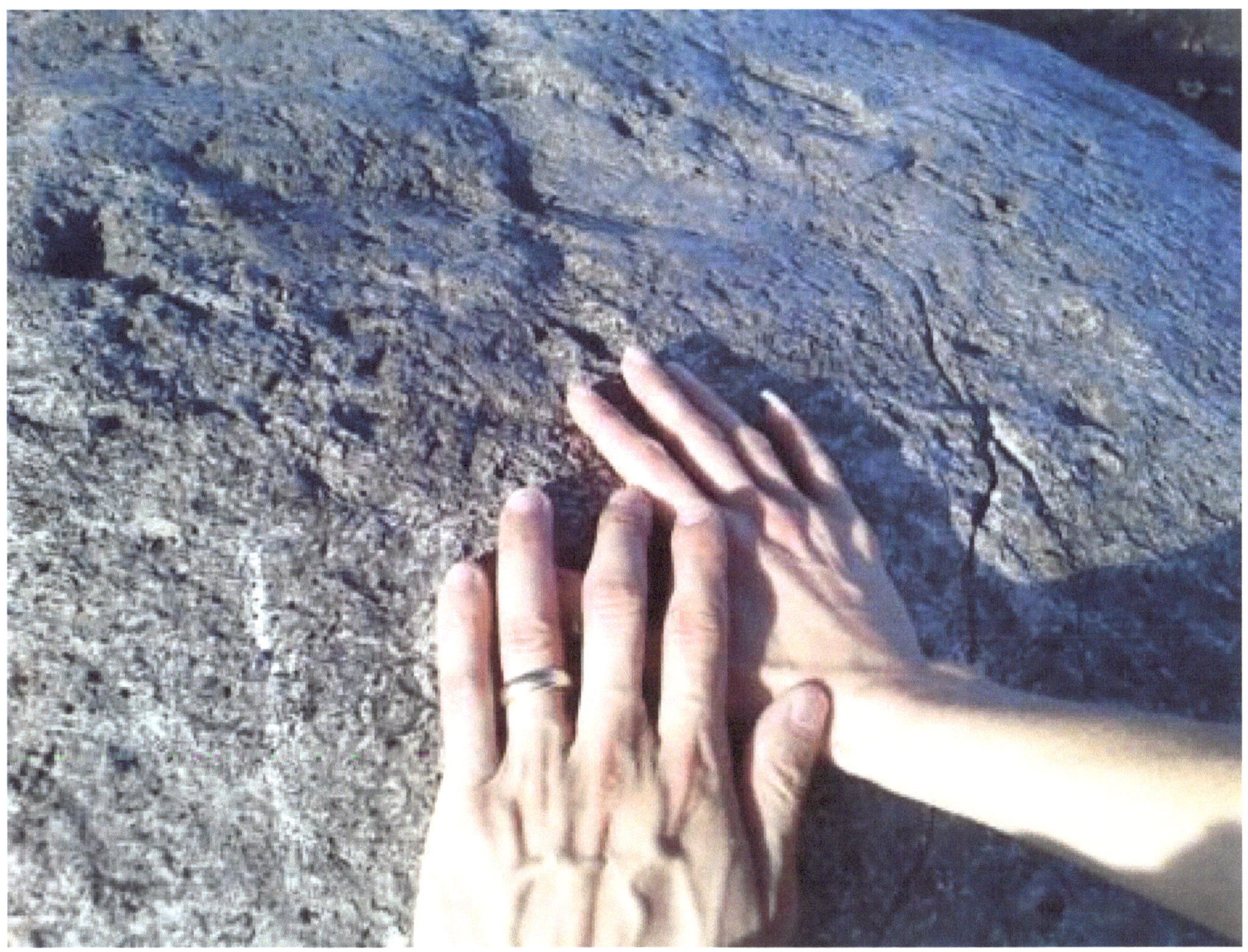

Me and Rocky in 2009!

I slowed down, limiting myself to jogging with a friend and taking walk breaks. I did a 5K race with my husband (and walk breaks), only to collapse in a seizure immediately afterward. Then after going for about a year seizure-free, we decided to give 5K-ing another try. A mile or so into the race…I went down, convulsing.

So now, even though I'm neuro-drugged to the max, I'm back to walking. I carry bags for the litter and recyclables I pick up along the way, and I enjoy saying hi to passers-by. I marvel at the beauty of nature, even as I mourn my running days.

But who am I to complain? I know what it is to be housebound and worse from a TBI and broken body. I know the feeling of constant drowsiness, the confusion, the loss of control of your own life. In lesser ways, I'm still dealing with all of that.

But it does get better, little by little. *Dooni dooni kononi be nyaga da,* as they say in Mali.

I live in northern Illinois, a very flat part of the country, but in my suburb there are a couple of hills besides the one I used as my running course. When I climb to the top of either one, I can see Rocky, miles away, and I always give my old friend a (quiet) shout-out.

You know how Sylvester Stallone's character ran up those steps while training in the original movie? Maybe I'm tough like that…so just maybe that boulder isn't only the goal; maybe I *am* Rocky. Mind you, I wouldn't hurt a fly, but 29 years ago, I had a summer newspaper copy-editing internship in Philadelphia, and the whole group of us "word nerds" did the triumphant "Rocky" run up those actual steps.

To those still struggling up the Mountain, never forget: *Dooni dooni kononi be nyaga da.*

Meet Lisa Yee

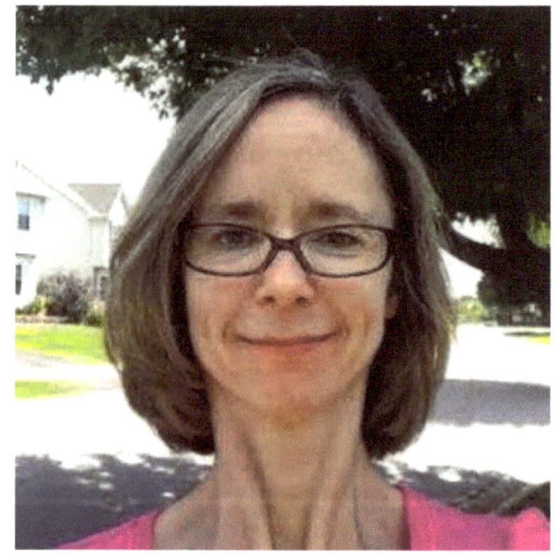

Lisa Yee of suburban Chicago suffered a traumatic brain injury/epilepsy in a 2008 car accident. Before her injury, she had been a newspaper editor for two decades after graduating from the Indiana University School of Journalism. It was there she met her husband, Ted. They have a daughter, Megan, of Chicago.

Post TBI, Lisa became certified as a yoga instructor and now volunteers teaching yoga at a women's shelter and a veteran's center.

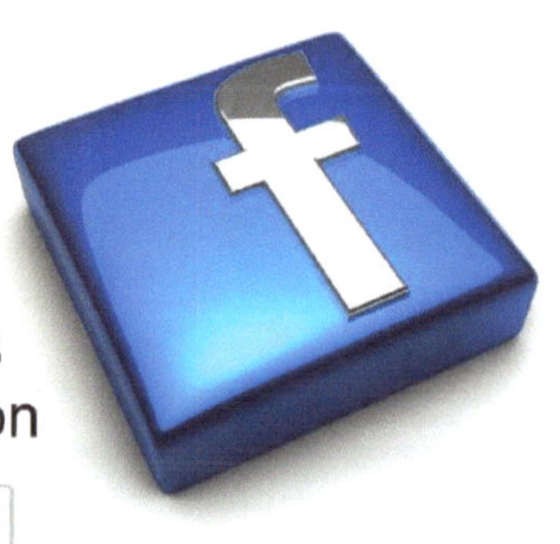

Finding Senior Housing can be complex, but it doesn't have to be.

Call A Place for Mom. Our Advisors are trusted, local experts who can help you understand your options. Since 2000, we've helped over one million families find senior living solutions that meet their unique needs.

"You can trust **A Place for Mom** to help you."

– Joan Lunden

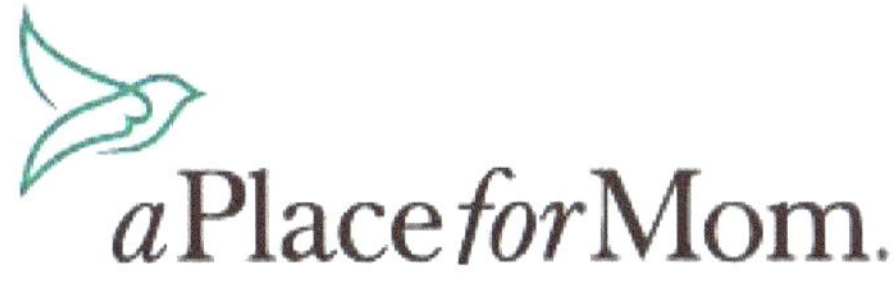

A Free Service for Families.
Call: (844) 578-9504

A Place for Mom is the nation's largest senior living referral information service.
We do not own, operate, endorse or recommend any senior living community.
We are paid by partner communities, so our services are completely free to families.

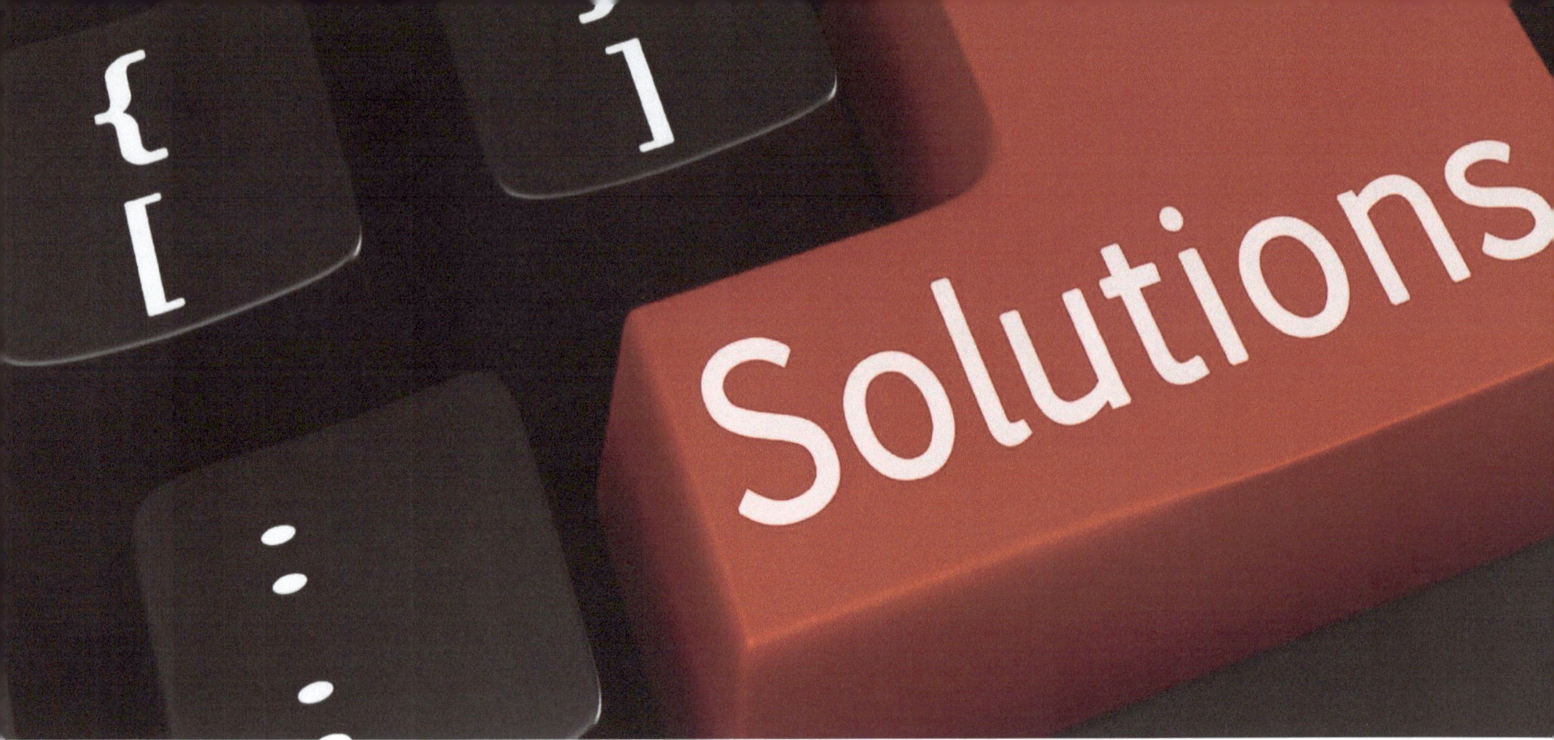

We Need Solutions

By Jeff Sebell

After we experience a brain injury we want answers to some important questions: when will I be my old self again, and how do I get myself back?

Unfortunately, there are no answers.

We learn quickly that, much to our dismay, there is no roadmap for life after brain injury. There is no schedule. There is no "approved method" for living. The best we can do is listen to doctors and therapists, as well as other survivors who have already travelled this road, hoping we can find ways to improve and live a fulfilled life.

> "We learn quickly that, much to our dismay, there is no roadmap for life after brain injury."

The path to achieve some sort of "normalcy" in our lives is tedious and frustrating; filled with failure and emotional turmoil. We are haunted by how our lives have changed and by the upheaval we live in daily, and we look for ways we can make our lives work.

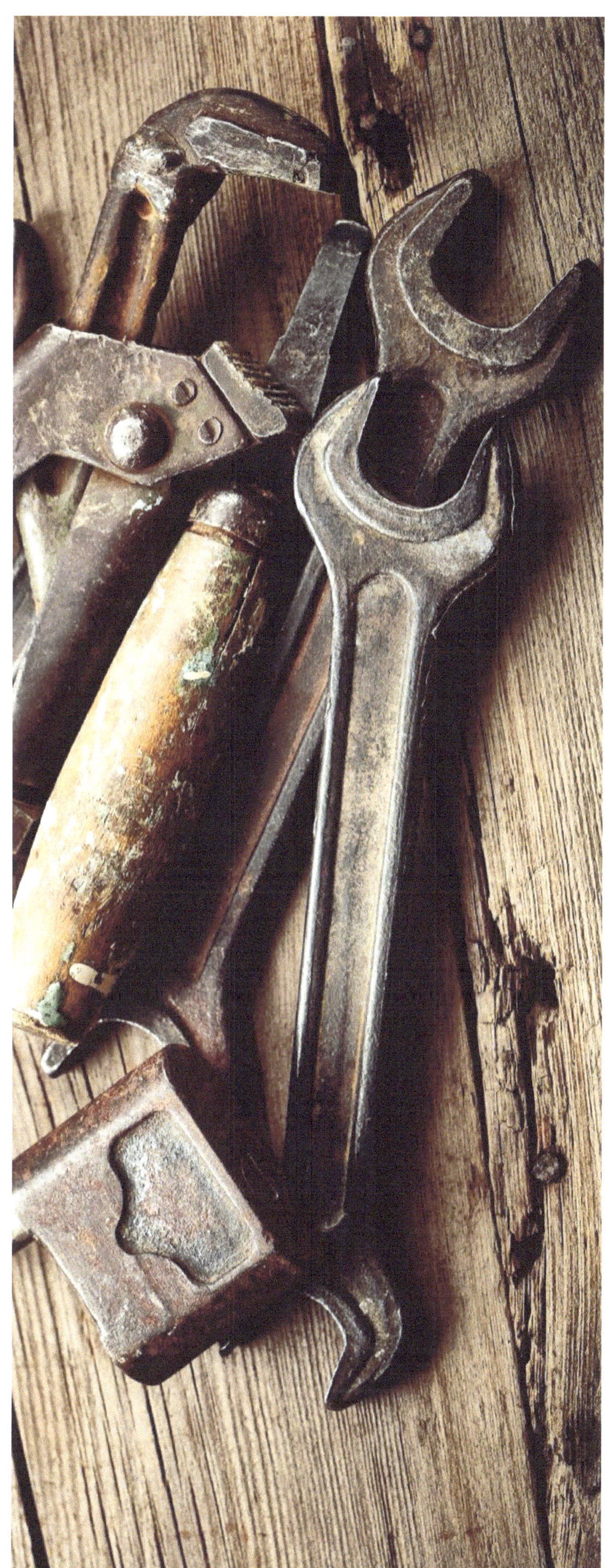

And That Method Is...

Insightful survivors have been able to employ the use of "strategies" which allow them to function better on a daily basis. An example of a simple strategy is this: in order to combat forgetfulness, one might leave things lying around so they are visible and, and this way, make one less apt to forget about them.

I'm sure that each of us can think of similar routines we have developed that allow us to be successful in different situations.

As you can deduce from this example, or might know from your own personal experience, one needs all kinds of strategies for all types of situations; meaning there is an infinite number of strategies that one must employ in daily life. Ultimately, we become a repository for these "strategies"; human beings who sometimes spend more time thinking and planning about how to go about our lives than actually living.

These "strategies", although beneficial, are really not what might be called *solutions*. They are *tools*, or *workarounds* that allow us to get by. They are used as any tool might be used: we have to stop and think about what tool to use and how to use it. We don't really act on impulse or instinct because it is not **us** that is solving the problem. It is the use of the tool.

Let me show you an example:

Imagine you are trying to start your lawnmower but it is broken and you need a part. In order to mow your lawn without losing time, you devise something that takes the place of the right part so the machine can work until you are able to purchase the part and fix the lawnmower. That is an example of a "strategy" that is not really a solution; it is a temporary fix.

Relying On Strategies

Using strategies shows you have the ability to improvise in life, and it is absolutely normal and good to employ strategies to make things work so you can be successful. We want to do things in a way that makes us feel capable, as though we are a functioning part of society again, performing near or at the level we used to.

When we talk about strategies, we speak of things that are *helpful in achieving a goal*, but are not cures. Strategies are tools we use to get us through the day.

Now, think about this: ideally, do we really want to spend our whole lives having to think about and implement strategies for every situation we find ourselves in? I'm sure we would all rather be able to react and achieve our goals naturally.

What Can We Do?

Concentrating on strategies as a way to be successful in life distracts us from the true mission, which is to regain and live our life as a human being, not a person who lives from activity to activity and strategy to strategy. Although strategies are an important part of life after brain injury, what we are really looking for are *solutions*. Finding *solutions* is difficult and frustrating, but necessary. Otherwise we become dependent on strategies for every situation, rather than looking for ways for us to react instinctually, without taking the time and energy to think and plan.

Where do we even begin to look for these solutions?

You Are the Solution

It is easy to become reliant on strategies when the real goal should be weaning ourselves off them. When we become reliant on strategies and

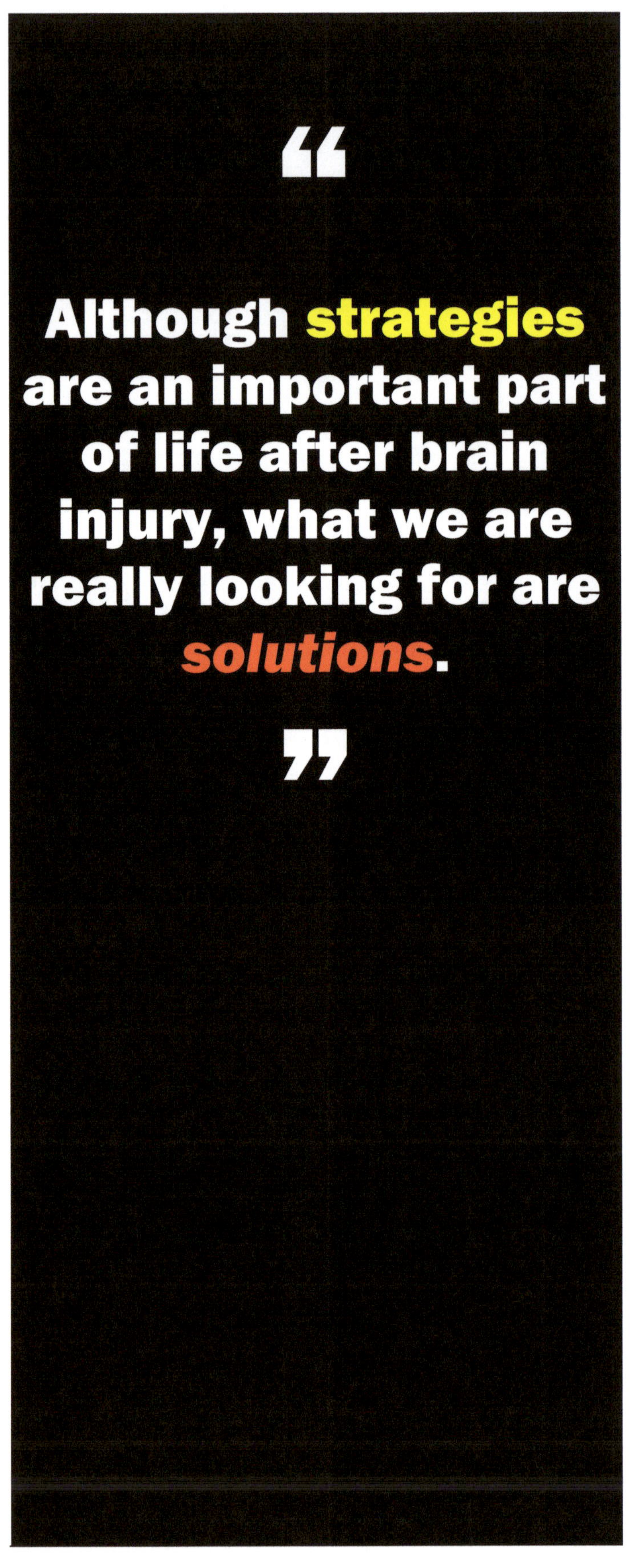

treat them as solutions rather than "work-arounds" we run the danger of not thinking "outside the box" and not moving forward in our life and we all want to progress and be strong individuals. Weaning ourselves off strategies and looking for solutions, as much as possible, involves looking at the bigger picture, trusting ourselves and knowing ourselves so we are able to handle ourselves in different situations.

We certainly need strategies, but we also need an elastic approach to life after brain injury where we treat ourselves as humans, humans who might make mistakes but who try to figure out a better way to do things. To do this we need to learn about ourselves: about what makes us tick, about what drives us as people, and we need to learn how to be who we have become after our brain injury. If we develop a better understanding of ourselves, accepting our situation, perhaps over time we can learn to trust ourselves without having to be as reliant on strategies.

Meet Jeff Sebell

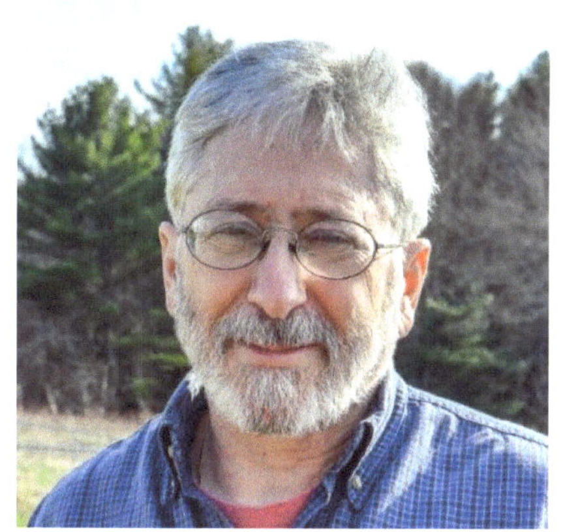

Jeff Sebell is a published Author, Speaker and Blogger writing about Traumatic Brain Injury and the impacts of his own TBI which he suffered in 1975 while attending Bowdoin College. He has been active in the community since the inception of the NHIF and was on the founding board of directors of the MA chapter. His book "Learning to Live with Yourself after Brain Injury," was released in August of 2014 by Lash Publishing.

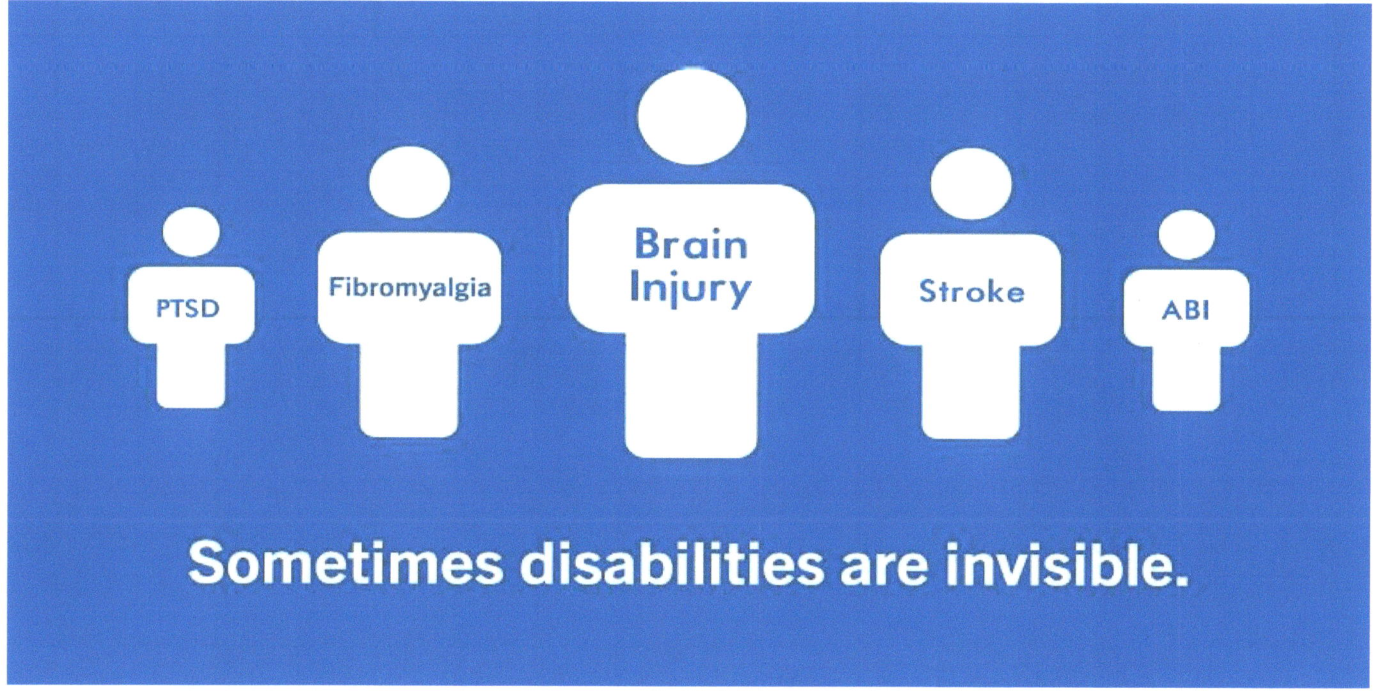

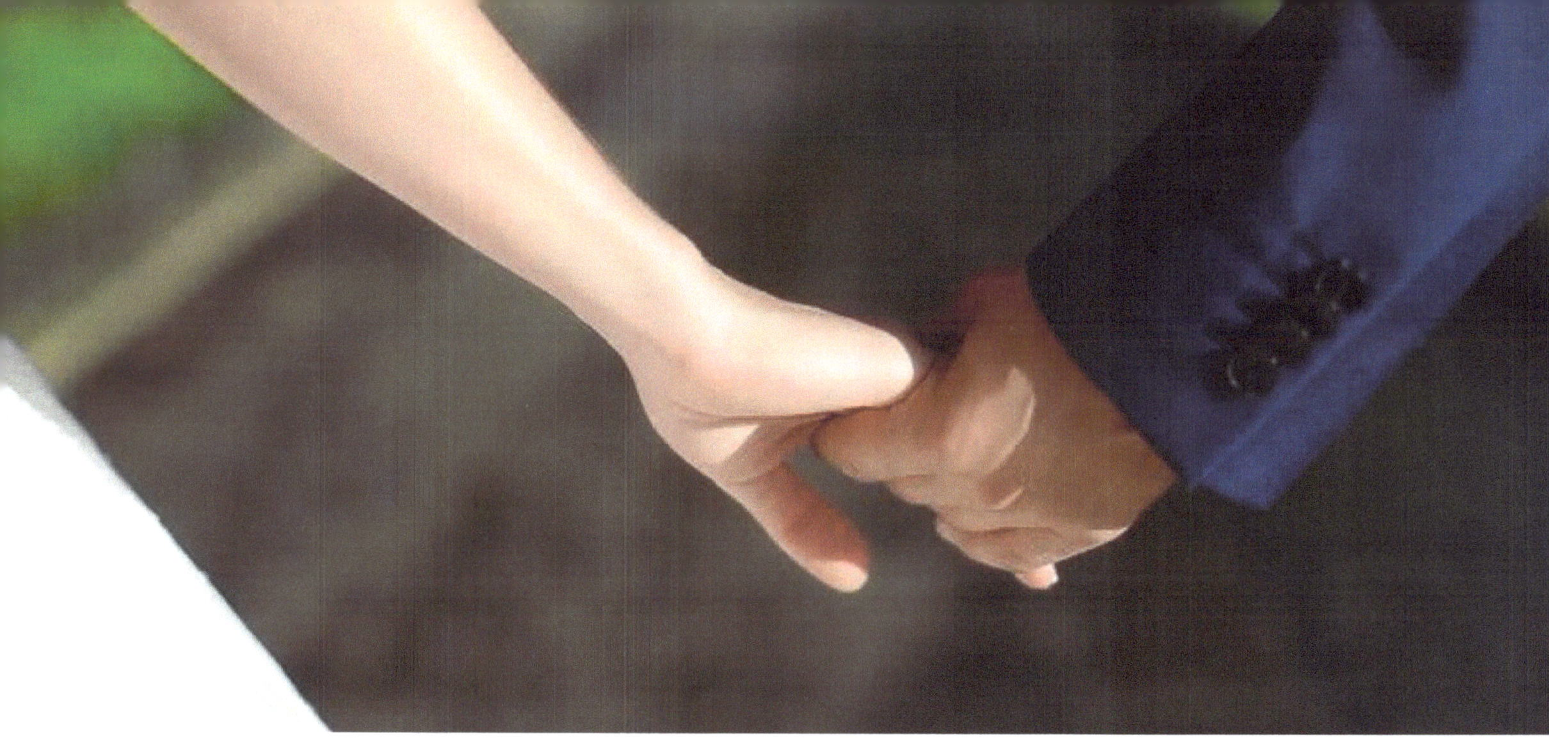

My Wedding Day

By Christina Riley

I could hardly believe it. The event that I had anticipated had finally arrived. The morning of my wedding was non-stop. My appointments were all in place, with reminders set on my cell phone. My short-term memory limits my ability to recall new information, like that of specific times. Reminders are my way of dealing with my memory loss.

I had to be sure that everything was ready by the time the limo came to the house to pick up me and my bridal party. Thankfully, I received a confirming text from each of my bridesmaids the night before. They all knew about my memory challenges.

It was helpful for me to have the texts to refer to during the morning of my wedding. My mother was there to help me with everything that morning. She helped to keep my nerves under control.

"Looking back at all of the monumental decisions I had to make, choosing my gown was the biggest one."

Looking back at all of the monumental decisions I had to make, choosing my gown was the biggest one. I recall going to the bridal store with my mother. We were surrounded by a seemingly infinite number of gowns. I knew the style I wanted. I just had to be sure that I could handle our trip to the store. Mobility is a limiting factor of my brain injury.

My dream of a "mermaid" style gown would only work if I could move in it. Since my injury, I now tend to walk with a wider stance, trying to hold my balance in place while transferring my weight back and forth. The first gown we decided to try on proved to be too tight around my legs. The next one, much to my relief, was perfect. Around mid-thigh, the silk belled out, achieving the mermaid style I wanted. There also was more give to the fabric. Luckily, I found the gown of my dreams, which for most brides is a battle of its own.

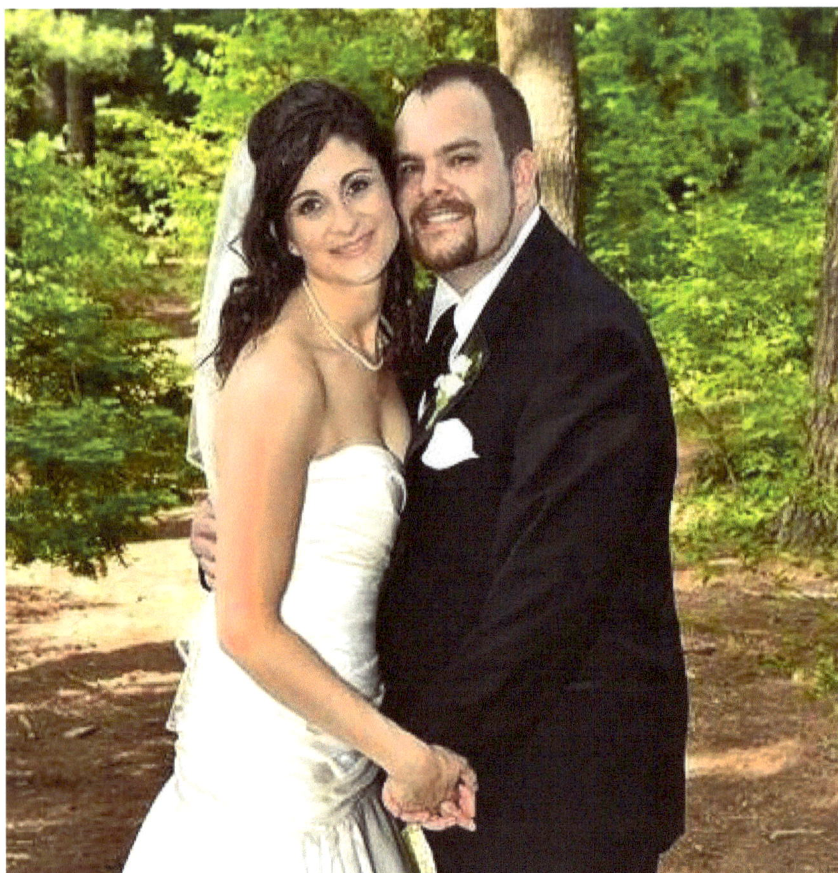

My next challenge proved to be the shoes that would accompany my gown. I have always had narrow feet, so I needed to find a shoe that would stay on my foot. As is most apparent, I also have an inhibited walking ability. The style had to be flat, without a heel. The shoe store we went to had a very limited variety of flats. I found a pearl white, almost lacy mesh-type of ballet flat.

There was an issue with the width of these flats, specifically in the toe area. I needed the shoe to be tighter, securing my foot so my heel would not pop out when I walked, which would ultimately hamper my stability. My mother, my right-hand woman in this quest, thought of a foam mesh material we could place under my toes, adding to the shoe. The shoe problem was now solved thanks to my mom.

So many decisions led up to that wonderful day. There were so many details. From dresses, to the church, to the reception, as well as having numerous details being discussed and determined, wedding planning is a lot of work. The secret to remembering all this complete madness was in a small feature in my cell phone. Under the "Notes" section of my phone, I had a section called "Wedding." This is where I kept all the final wedding details. I listed the date, the church, the priest, my bridesmaids and groomsmen, possible reception venues (until we decided of course), and the times and details for my hair and makeup to be done on the actual day.

This became very handy when I was speaking to someone about my wedding and couldn't recall a certain detail. Final plans, in black and white, were added to this section, always there for me to pull up, when I couldn't confidently remember something.

My wedding day had finally arrived. A reminder let me know that the stylist that was coming to do my hair and I had a picture of the style I wanted in my inbox. I could not forget that, as I wanted it just right. After having my hair done, it was time for my makeup. Now two checks were off my list.

Suddenly, the last of my bridesmaids arrived, just as the reminder on my cell went off to let me know, "Bethany will be a little late." At this point, with the help of my handy reminders, I knew all was on track to be the happiest day of my life. Now all that was on my mind was the walk down that aisle, with my father of course, approaching my husband to be. The joyous exhilaration of this moment that was to come brought tears to my eyes as we all got into the limo.

I like to share the stories of my life to motivate people never to give up on their struggles, whatever they may be. Everyone has challenges. If you stay positive and optimistic, recovery from a traumatic brain injury means that you are always changing and improving. Planning my wedding reminded me that anything is possible!

Meet Christina Riley

Christina writes…

"I have always been a hard worker, in all that I do. After being hit by a car while crossing a street in front of my school, my life was literally thrown upside down. After waking up from a two-week coma, I was at square one. I had to relearn how to walk, needing to wear plastic inserts in my shoes, keeping my feet in the flexed position. My left arm was also greatly immobilized, now being very tight and slow to move. My short-term memory is tremendously impacted. I have never stopped trying to overcome my challenges. Because of this tenacious attitude, I am where I am at today!"

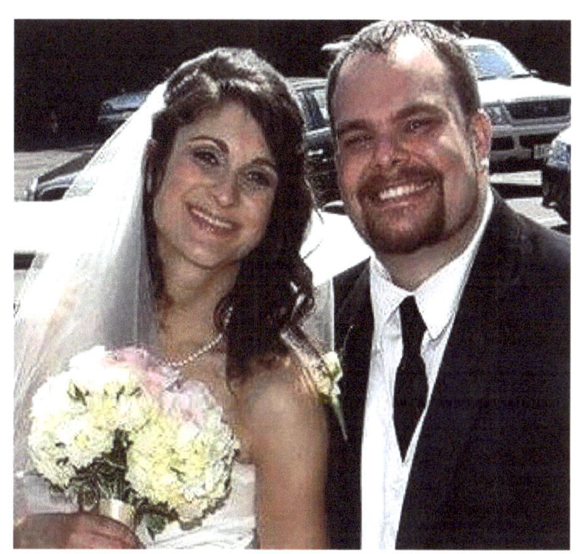

"My strength lies solely in my tenacity."
- Louis Pasteur

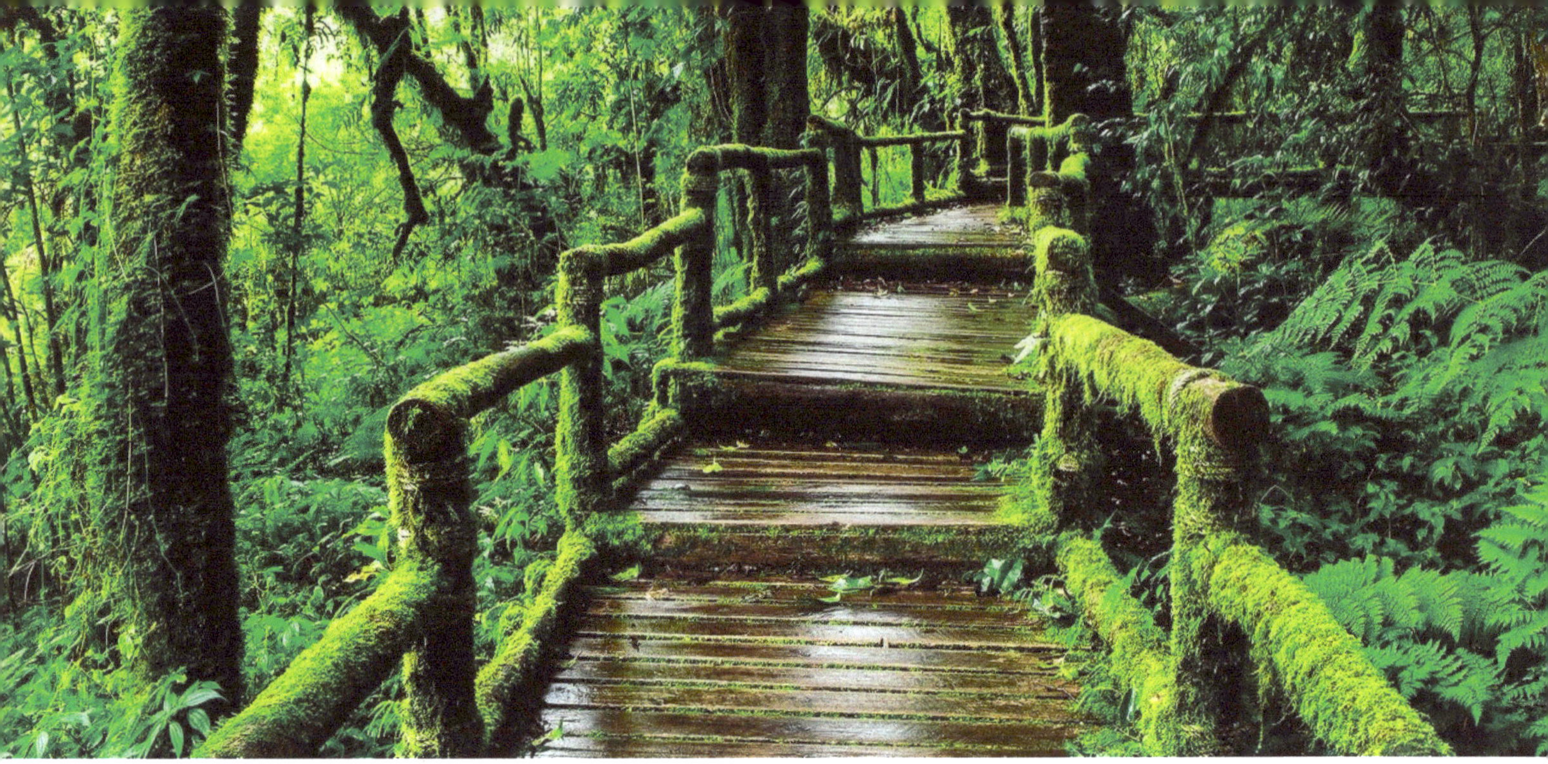

The Need for Compassion

By Katy Austin

A few years ago, my cousin Tobie sustained a traumatic brain injury. I affectionately referred to her as my "sistercuz." This is a term of endearment. In many ways, I have learned that focusing on how her brain injury happened does not help either her or me. I have also learned that moving forward and supporting her in the best way I know how, is a lifelong journey.

I have some prior experience as a caregiver of loved ones. While I do not consider myself an expert, I do try to be mindful about what I do, what I say, and how I support those close to me. Dealing with the injured, sick, or someone with a disability has some common ground, but not necessarily common sense. I am hoping that sharing my experience helps someone else to develop compassion and understanding.

There are a few things that I have learned not to do. I do not disregard or diminish how someone feels on any given day.

> "I am hoping that sharing my experience helps someone else to develop compassion and understanding."

A seemingly innocent statement like, "You seem fine to me," can completely invalidate how your loved one feels. Post-injury or illness, how the person feels daily can vary widely. You may think verifying that they look all right is a compliment or testament to the hard work they are doing, but when they hear it they may feel that you are not hearing how they really feel.

When they are cranky or irritable, do not take it personally. There can be many things going on with the mind and body post injury or illness, and a whole lot of them may have nothing to do with you. I understand now that brain injury can foster depression and anxiety. It can fuel chronic pain and sleep disruptions. Healthy and uninjured people get grumpy under such conditions. A brain injury can compound things further. Just practice unconditional love and recognize the struggle.

Be patient, and when frustration arises, be patient AND kind. Over the years, I have seen some examples of caregivers who were not ideal. I recognize that I have fallen short when fatigue was plaguing me, or stress confounding me. Saying things like, "How many times do I have to tell you?" or, playing doctor and suggesting, "Your problem is….." is no help at all.

I see perfectly healthy people lose their stream of thought when overly tired, and the most organized persons still forget things or need to have people repeat something they did not hear the first time. I can

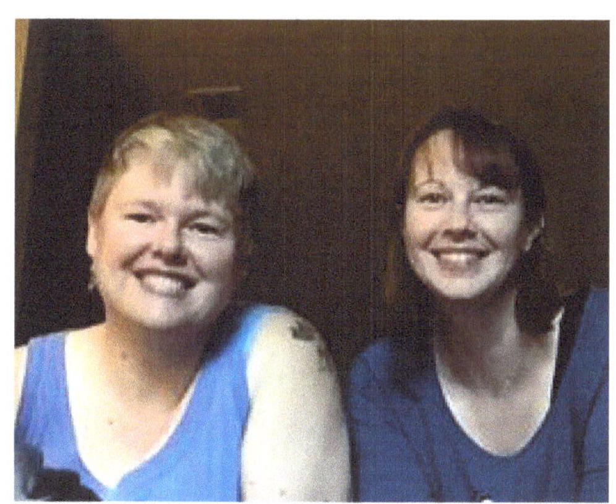

Katy and her "Sistercuz" Tobia

imagine how frustrating it would be to have your injured mind working against you and having to ask for information beyond what you used to need. Reacting to this frustration with further frustration helps no one.

Suggesting you might have better medical advice beyond the likely litany of specialists they have already seen borders on arrogance. In many ways, they do not need another medical professional in their lives; they need a friend, a sibling, a loved one. It's a different situation if you know they are seeking tips or suggestions, but unsolicited advice is often unrequired.

"Let me help." This one I still struggle with, as I am a problem solver by trade. I have a personality that wants to help others improve and succeed. Help isn't always helpful if you end up disempowering your loved one in the process. Watching a loved one fight or fail through physical therapy is no easy thing to witness, but sometimes simply bearing witness is the best love you can offer.

Doing the work for them doesn't help them rebuild. Lacking patience for how fast they may be moving on any given day does not help them regroup. Being available for when they ask for help is the best support one can offer.

My last piece of experience to share is also my own toughest to manage. It is very easy to be around the survivor in your life and feel they are lucky to be alive. While undoubtedly true, throwing "you're lucky to be alive," comments around without some background or context can inadvertently remind your loved one how unlucky they really feel.

Over time, I have learned that telling someone they are awesome, or that they rock, or that you love them, seems to go over well, any time.

Meet Katy Austin

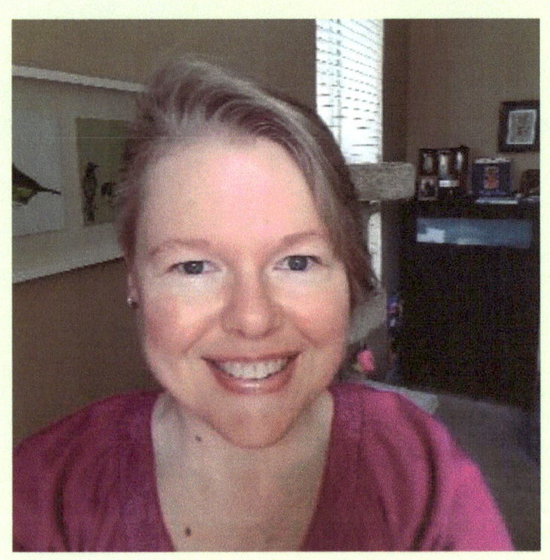

Katy loves reading, writing and motorcycling. For many years she cared for her life partner with AIDS, and today wants to support as best she can, her Sistercuz recovering from a grade three concussion with front left lobe damage and post-concussion syndrome with seizures.

Katy has learned through trial, error, and hard knocks that supporting someone involves learning what support looks like for that loved one through their eyes. Getting out of our own head and into a day in the life of someone with a brain injury is one of the hardest lessons to learn.

Things are never quite as scary when you've got a best friend.

~Bill Watterson

What is TBI?
By Tiffany Gross

TBI.
What is it?
Well, I know what it is not. It is not you.
It should not be who you are. It does not define you.
It should only be a part of you.
You are not TBI.
You have a TBI.
It is not you.
You are not it.
You have a name, and it is not TBI.
You have a personality separate from this disability.
You are who you are because of you.
Not because of your TBI.
When you introduce yourself you do not say,
"Hi, my name is TBI."
If you do, stop it!
You come first, you hear me?

Meet Tiffany Gross

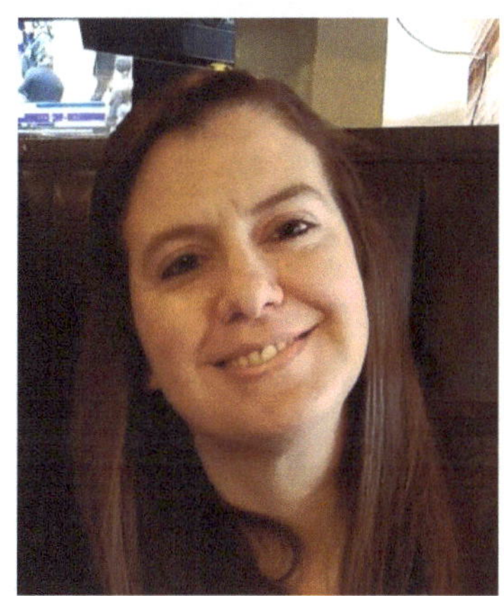

Tiffany wrote this poem with her friend Marvin. She writes…

"Marvin Tibbs and I have been writing poetry together over the years. His car accident happened in October of 2014. We have been working together and trying to enjoy ourselves as much as we can while on this TBI journey. We both have found that writing has been helpful in the healing process."

Promise me you'll always remember: You're braver than you believe, and stronger than you seem, and smarter than you think. ~A.A. Milne

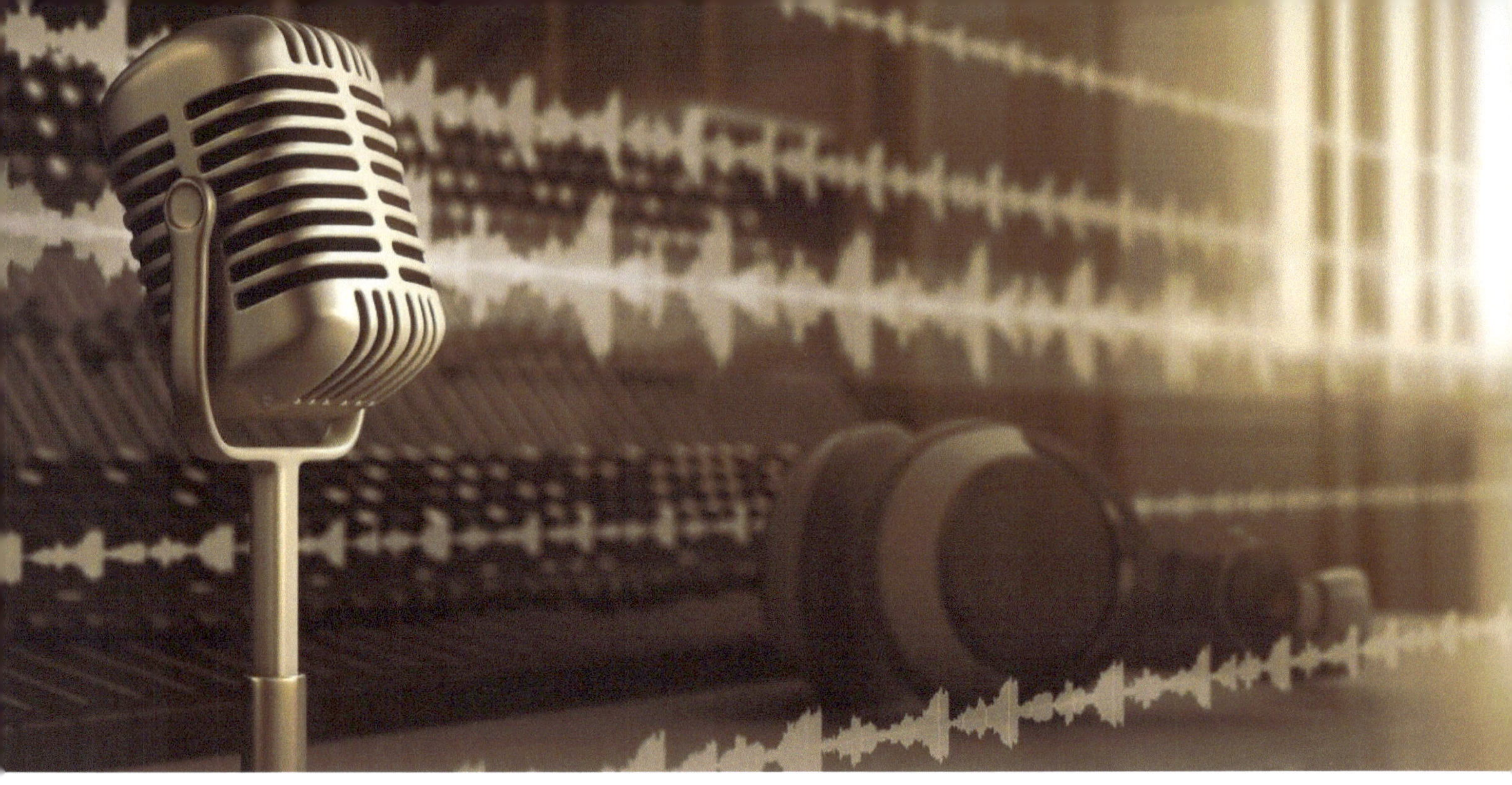

Changing the Inner Narrative

By David A. Grant

We've all got it, that inner voice that constantly narrates our lives.

Stumble in public, and most of us hear the same thing, "I hope nobody saw that!" Speed past a police officer well above the posted speed limit and that inner voice becomes a bit more urgent, "Maybe he didn't see me," or, "Not another speeding ticket!"

Having our life narrated often keeps us safe from harm and can validate our choices on a day-to-day basis. It is simply part of being human.

But as many of us know, brain injury can complicate things. Gone can be the ability to know intuitively when and how to handle things. Without warning, our inner narrator takes on a new power.

> "For many years, even while making significant gains in my brain injury recovery, my inner voice was not my friend."

For many years, even while making significant gains in my brain injury recovery, my inner voice was not my friend. Well-intentioned friends and family would tell me how great I was doing. I would smile and offer a courteous "Thank you," but I was not drinking the Kool-Aid.

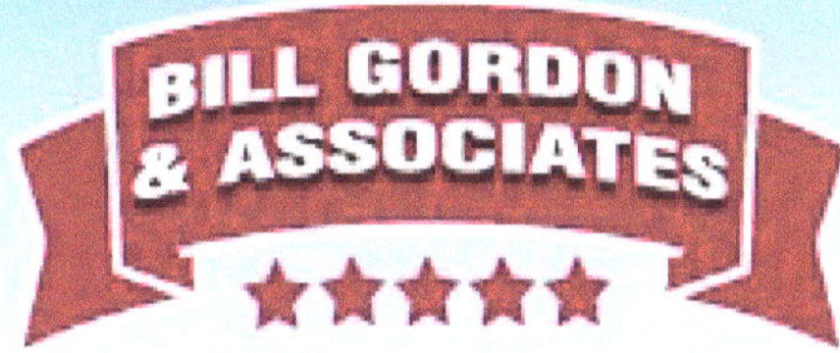
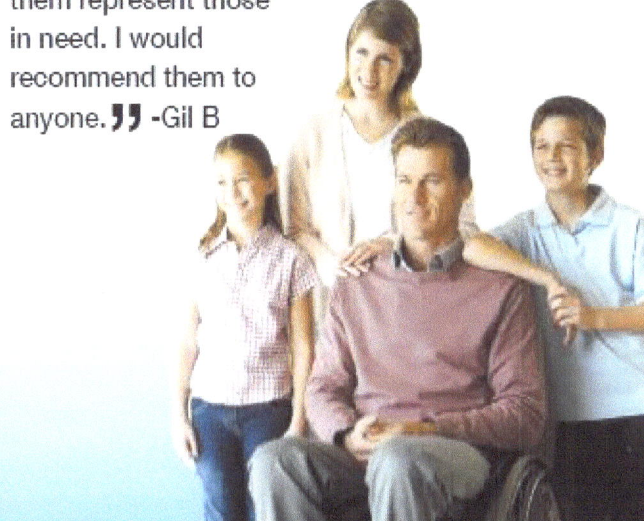

Not even close.

"You just want me to feel better. You don't mean that, and we both know it," sounded off the voice from deep within.

This was not an occasional experience. Almost daily, I was plagued with negative thoughts and a negative self-image. It was hard not to be. My words would simply give out when I was tired. My processing speed slowed to a snail's pace by 2:00 p.m. on most afternoons. Occasional vertigo often made me stumble.

Having these challenges at home alone is one thing, but being out in the world at large while compromised is not particularly conducive to a healthy self-image.

Sustaining a brain injury is the toughest thing I have ever experienced. There is no close second. I've had days that I wished that I never woke up, days thinking about how to end my life without devastating Sarah, and days where just drawing my next breath took a Herculean effort.

It should come as no surprise that negative thoughts were commonplace for me. The tragedy in all this is that I started to believe the lies I was telling myself.

"I'm never going to get any better."

"Life sucks, and then you die."

"I just can't do this anymore."

It was no way to live. Like a rudder steering a ship, my negative self-talk was steering me in the wrong direction. It was stealing the joy from my days and making what was already a heavy load to carry even heavier.

There was no real ah-ha moment when things changed. I just got tired of it. Negativity is exhausting.

Last year was a significant year in my recovery. I began sleeping better, my memory lapses were less frequent, and I began to string together longer stretches of good days. I began to feel more alive than I had in many years.

At some point, I decided to replace "I can't" with "I can, and I WILL!"

It was no overnight process. I began to listen, really listen, to my ongoing inner monologue. When negativity tried to creep in, I would immediately try to replace it with something positive. This took effort on my part, but it has already shown to be effort well spent.

Case in point: I can have two back-to-back tough TBI days. On one day, if the inner monologue leans toward the negative, it is a fast track to a bad day. Take a similar day and wrap positive thinking around it, a bad day becomes tolerable, and in some cases, it becomes a good day.

I don't kid myself for one moment. I will always have challenges because of my brain injury. You cannot wish away occasional speech problems. Positive self-talk will not take away neuro-fatigue. While I am forever changed by my brain injury, I steadfastly refuse to be reduced by it.

I cannot change what happened to me, but I can change my perceptions and my outlook. Choosing to focus on the positive inner narrative makes me feel better. And in the end, isn't that a big part of what brain injury recovery is all about, feeling better?

Meet David A. Grant

David A. Grant is a freelance writer based out of southern New Hampshire and the publisher of HOPE Magazine. He is the author of Metamorphosis, Surviving Brain Injury.

He is also a contributing author to Chicken Soup for the Soul, Recovering from Traumatic Brain Injuries. David is a BIANH Board Member. David is a regular contributing writer to Brainline.org, a PBS sponsored website.

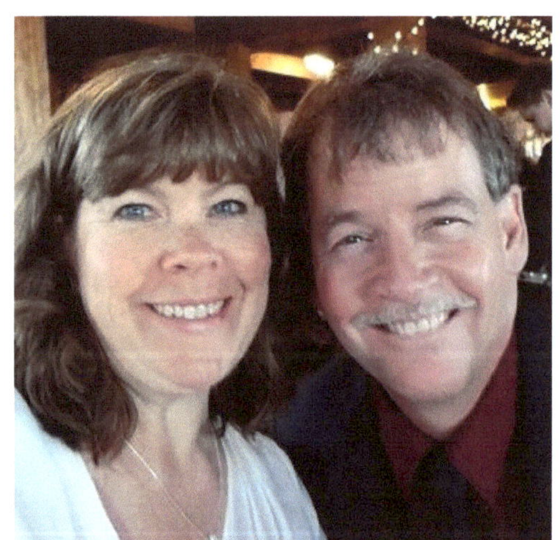

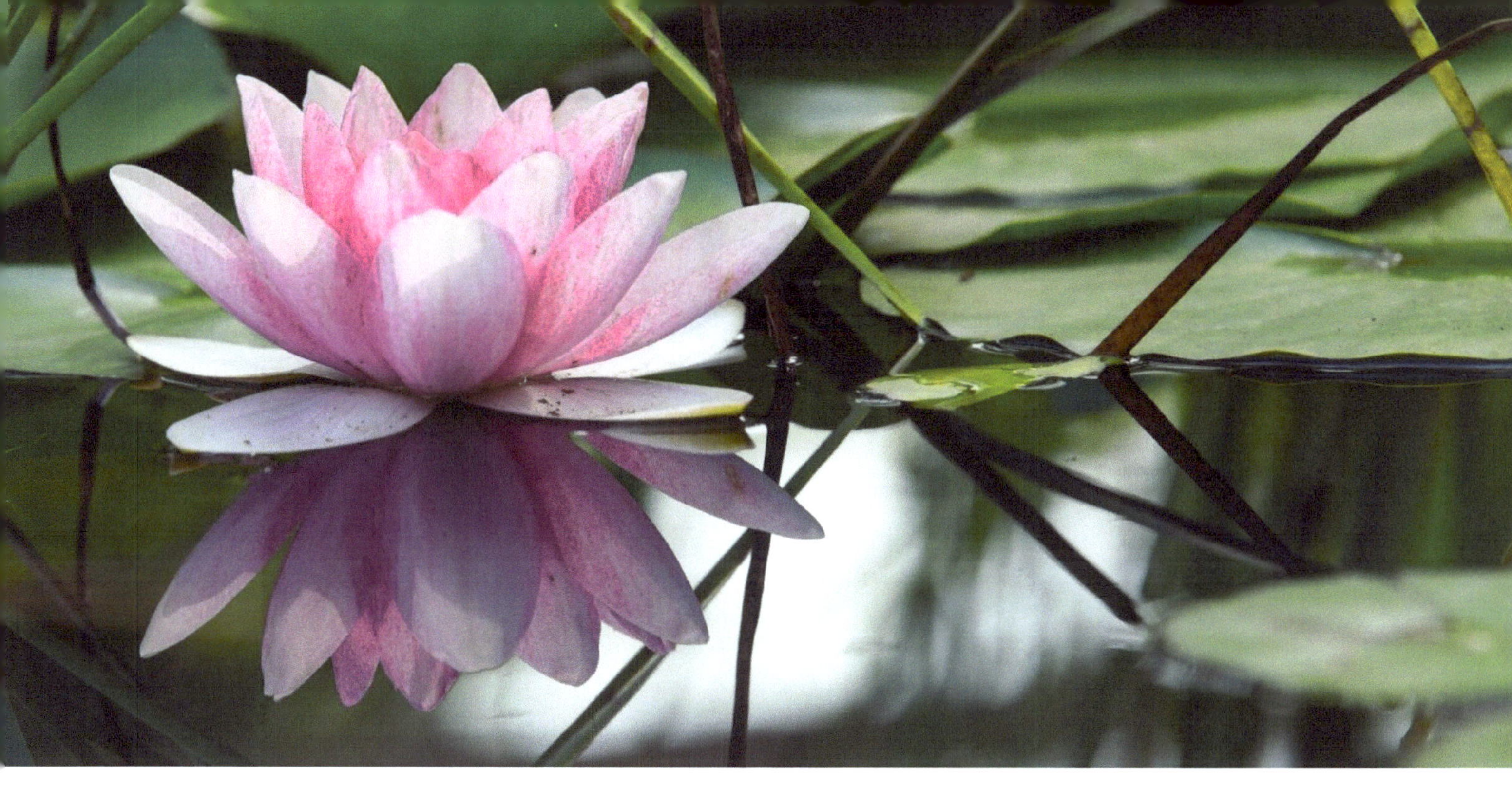

I Am Still Healing

By Mary Underwood

Today, I'm a single mom looking after my elderly parents as best I can. I had been the primary caregiver and breadwinner for three generations going from an annual six figure income to nothing. My son is now twenty-two and in college and my parents are eighty-nine and eighty-four. I am forty-six years old.

My health issues began when I incurred the first of six head/brain injuries, at work, on July 12, 2005. Our acting Team Lead was horse-playing in the office and hit me on the left side of my head just above my ear with a ball he had thrown at a fellow coworker. I did not see it coming. That injury also created a secondary arachnoid cyst on my brain behind my left eye at the front of my left temporal lobe, due to the whiplash effect, along with focal and diffuse brain injuries.

> "I couldn't be around my son playing or going to his basketball games anymore because I was sensitive to light."

My endocrine system was disrupted causing LOTS of effects, hair growth on my face, abnormal balding pattern, my hair went completely gray by age thirty-six, and reduced taste and smell. I couldn't be around my son playing or going to his basketball games anymore because I was sensitive to light. I had slurred speech, tiredness, and coordination issues; I lost function on the right side of my body three separate times and still have numbness and swelling when fatigued, brain fog and headaches. There is nothing about me that has not been affected by these injuries.

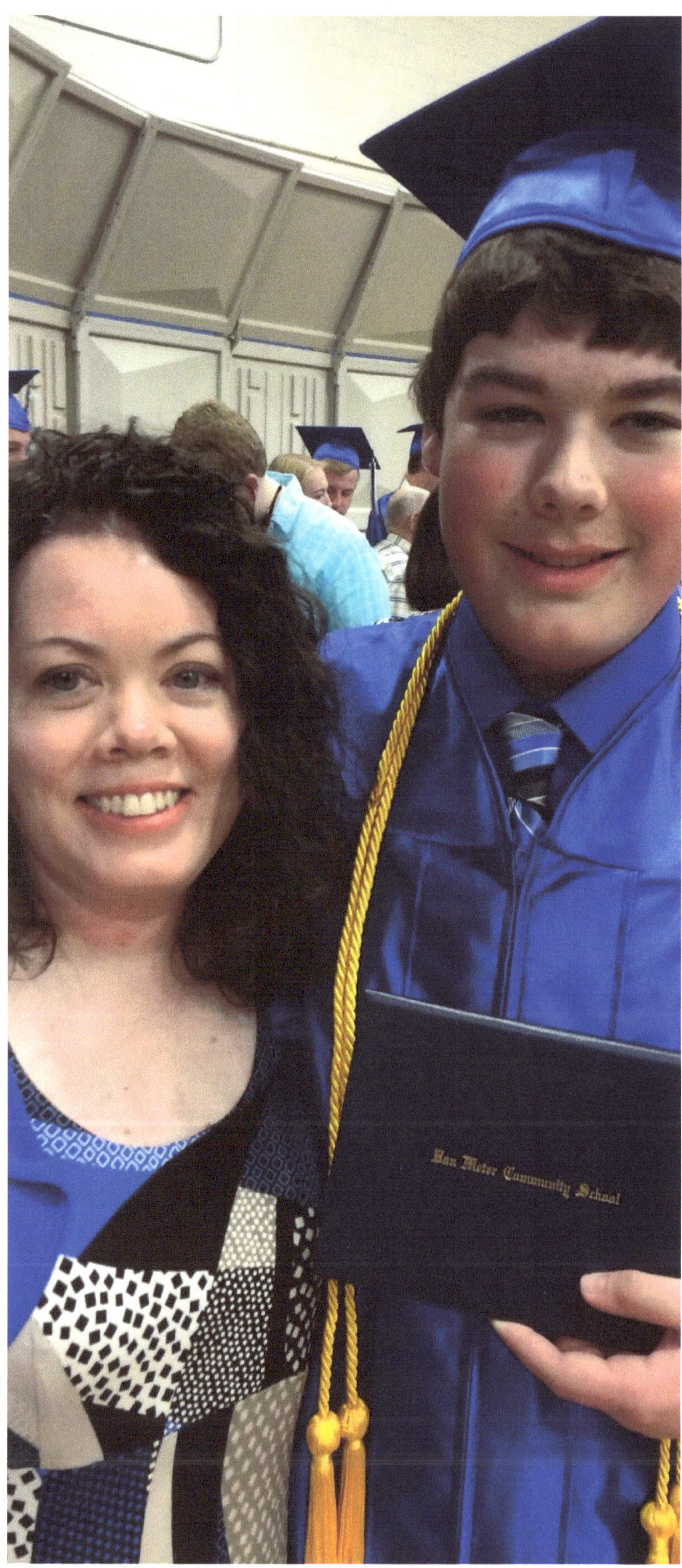

I had two brain surgeries at Cedars Sinai Medical Center, in 2008. During the second one, the surgeon nicked a vein causing a hemorrhage and physical damage to my frontal and temporal lobes, along with causing encephalomalacia (softening and loss of brain tissue) in those areas of my brain. He also cut through my left trigeminal nerve and jaw muscle.

My car was rear-ended in 2012, on my way home from work. The driver hit me so hard that the back bumper was broken in half. I had whiplash, concussion and injuries to my neck and spine. Then, in November of 2013, I fell on the ice leaving work one day. I had landed in the parking lot with my left leg folded under me causing a pelvic joint injury. My car was rear-ended again in August of 2014, at a stop sign, and then had a fall on our front cement porch in February of 2016.

I am still dealing with PCS symptoms today, with neuro-fatigue being the catalyst for the cascade of my other symptoms, including headaches, dizziness, nausea, weakness, difficulty walking, blood pressure increase, body temperature decrease, shivering, shaking, ringing in my ears, and swelling in my mouth and throat. I continue to have cognitive issues as well, including memory and recall issues. Stress wears me out quickly, along with cognitive exertion and physical exertion.

I have had some improvements after HBOT therapy, like less anxiety, I'm happier, I have more energy, some of the reflexes on my left arm have returned. I have had better sleep as well. When I am able to sleep, I am no longer a morning person and I need ten to twelve hours of leep to feel rested. I'm hoping I'm still healing.

I've been through two rounds of neuro-rehabilitation using PT, SLT, and OT. They've helped. The neuropsychologist and his testing don't explain my loss of functioning energy-wise, with the cascade of PCS symptoms, nor the continued cognitive issues I have in my daily life. I've taken those tests so many times that I've memorized some of the answers, especially in the math portion.

My previous neuropsychologist said that doctors can get frustrated with people who are "very bright," because the neuropsych tests cannot gauge well the extent of injury we have. My IQ is up three points to 120 since my last testing when it was 117. That was after five injuries. I'm wondering what my starting IQ was. I know my language skills have diminished too and I still have word finding issues and words that come out wrong. I have to reread my emails too, to correct grammar and spelling which had not been a problem at all prior to the 2005 injury. I believe the HBOT treatments have helped me improve, but they are expensive and not affordable for me today.

> ## "I know my language skills have diminished too and I still have word finding issues and words that come out wrong."

Brain injury is no joke to endure. Every person is different, and every injury is different and every healing is different. Just because people don't bother to understand it, doesn't mean they cannot help to do something about it. There are healing options and there are rehabilitation methods that are more effective than others. We need to pursue healing and recovery and help those with brain injuries flourish, not just maintain them thinking that's just "good enough." There's always more possibility. Always. We need individualized care, period. And cutting edge. Think outside the box.

Meet Mary Underwood

Mary B Underwood is a 46 year-old college educated multiple brain injury survivor due to various accidents from 2005-2016. She's a single mom of a 22 year-old college student son and looks after her elderly parents as she is able to. She has had HBOT treatments with some objectively verified healing in 2015.

Her son Daniel has given her great purpose to keep seeking more healing and recovery from her injuries in order to hopefully flourish and thrive again one day to be the mom, daughter, sister, and friend she wants to be by continually pushing forward.

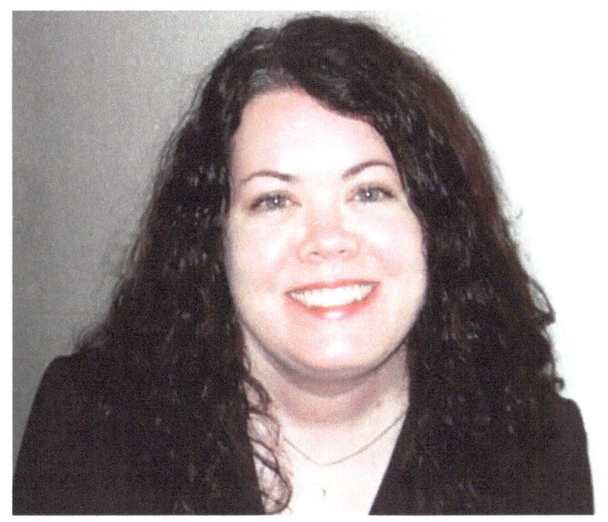

You've just read the fifty-first consecutive issue of HOPE Magazine. For close to four-and-a-half years, every month we have been able to bring you stories from survivors, caregivers, as well as members of the professional and medical community.

Over the years, we've had the honor to publish over 500 stories. Readers from around the world have reached out to us by email, some offering thanks and gratitude for HOPE Magazine, others asking to connect with specific contributors whose stories reflect their own.

There have been innumerable changes over the years as well. In early 2017, we made our publication available in print after hearing requests by readers for a print version. Last year's name change to a very simple *HOPE Magazine* allowed us to serve a larger brain injury community, as we shifted our focus from traumatic brain injury to brain injuries of all kinds – a change noted quite positively by our many stroke survivor readers.

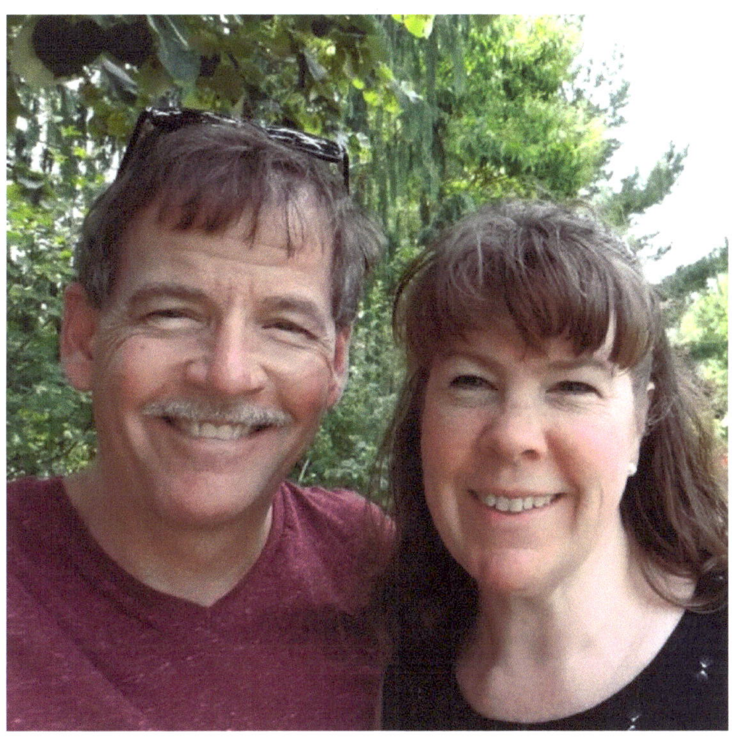

As we move forward, we will continue to listen to you and do all we can to honor the needs and wishes of the brain injury family.

If you have any suggestions as to how we can improve our publication, we'd love to hear from you. We take the time to read and reply to every email. In our community, opinion matters, and no one recovers alone.

We wish you all the best on your journey.

~David & Sarah